Nurse

by Ann-Marie Kishel

first step nonfiction

Lerner Publications Company · Minneapolis

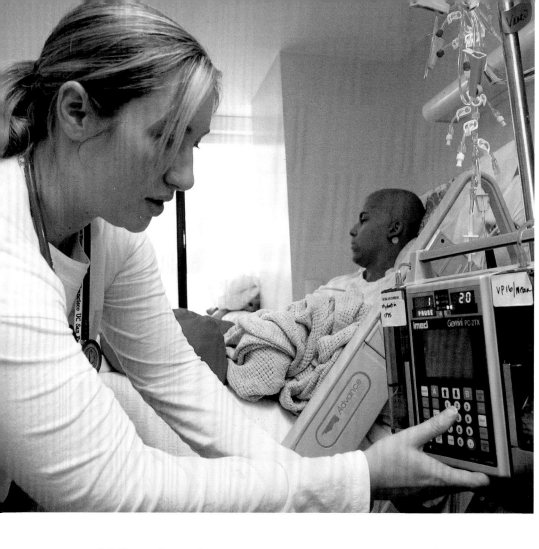

What does a nurse do?

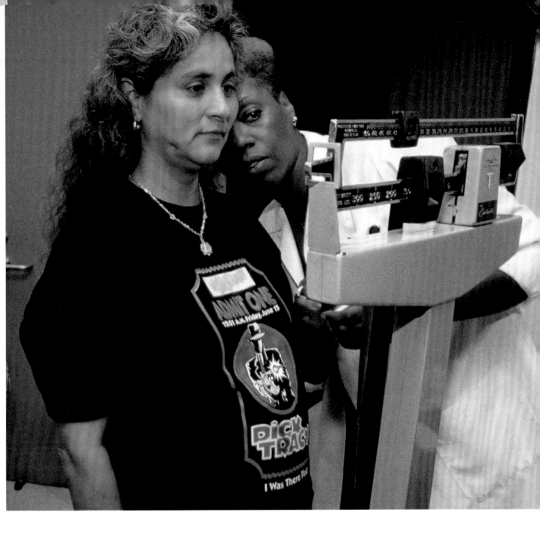

She weighs.

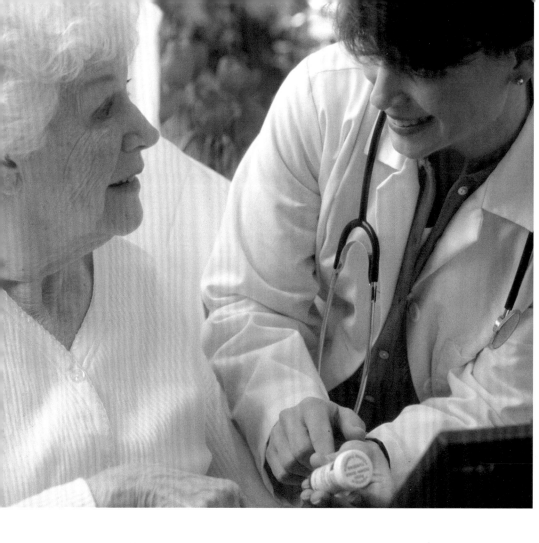

She gives medicine.

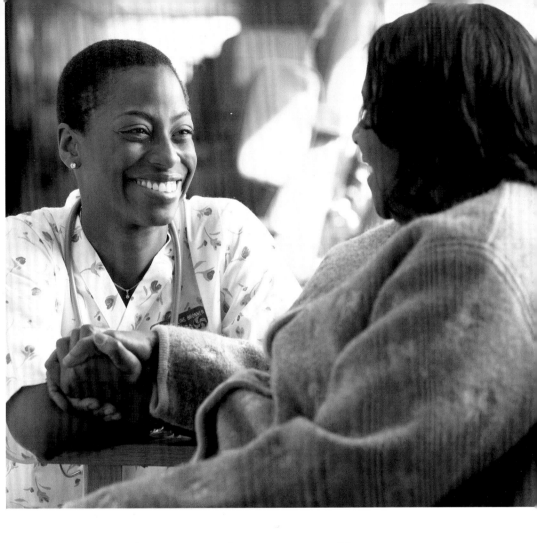

She asks questions.

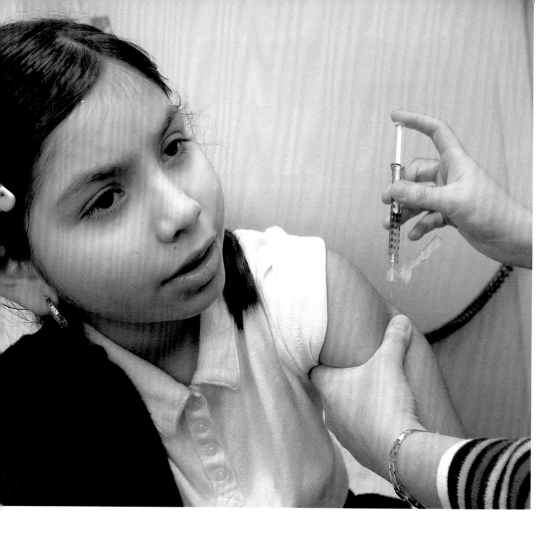

She gives shots.

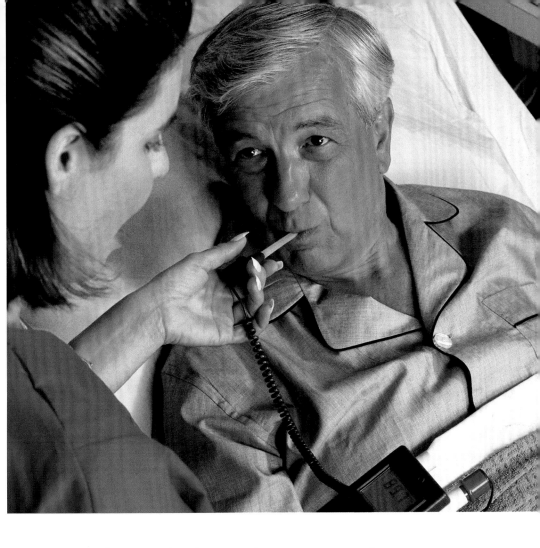

She takes temperatures.

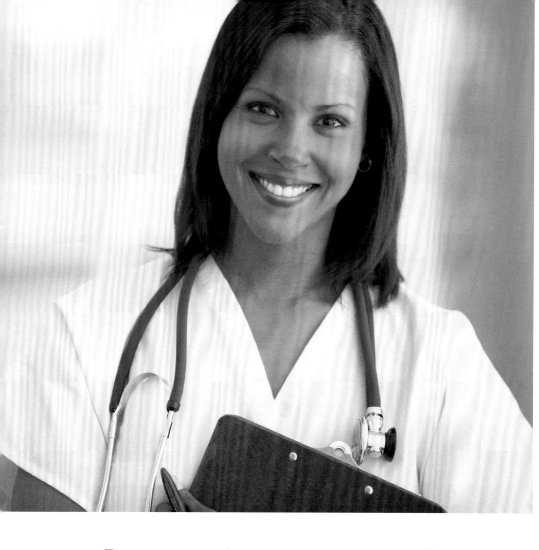

Do you know a nurse?